Get Hydrated for Life

Water is the secret ingredient.

Harmony Royce

DEDICATION

This book is especially for all those who yearn for life and wellness.

May it be a road map for your path to wellness and a source of motivating behaviors nourishing body and mind.

As you work for balance and well-being in your life, may wisdom and encouragement abound in every chapter.

CONTENTS

Disclaimers

This book's contents are meant for mainly general informative uses. Professional medical advice, diagnosis, or treatment is not meant to be replaced here. Regarding any health issues or illnesses, readers should speak with licensed medical professionals. The author and publisher disclaim all liability for any outcomes stemming from the use or abuse of anything included herein.

Craving for Positive Involvement

We truly hope this book helps you to better grasp hydration and motivates good lifestyle choices. Please get in touch with us personally should you have comments or questions. Your helpful comments are really valuable for our continuous efforts to raise standards and better serve our readers. Appreciate your understanding and support.

ACKNOWLEDGMENTS

I really want to thank everyone who helped to produce this book. This project is feasible thanks in great part to your support, ideas, and devotion. Particularly thanks to all of the writers, whose direction and knowledge was priceless all during the process.

CHAPTER 1

THE MEANING OF LIFE - REVEALING THE SIGNIFICANCE OF

WATER

1.1 Water: The Foundation of Our Health

Think of your body as a massive, intricate Lego set. Every Lego brick stands for a crucial component that your body requires in order to operate correctly. Water is one of the most crucial components of this set. Actually, an adult's body is composed of roughly 60% water, and that number rises for youngsters. That represents over 50% of you!

Every cell in your body contains water. It assists in delivering nutrients to your cells, which function as continuous little factories to maintain your health and vitality. Water aids in the body's waste removal process as well. Think of the water as the transportation system that keeps everything running smoothly and your cells as a busy city.

Your body releases water when you breathe, perspire, or use the restroom. That's why it's so crucial to consistently consume water. Should you fail to do so, your body may begin to experience thirst, an indication that your cells require additional water to function correctly. Your body requires water to function, much like an automobile needs gasoline.

1.2 Hydration's Evolution: From Ancient Knowledge to Contemporary Science

Water's significance has been understood by humans for thousands of years. Ancient societies, such as those in Mesopotamia and Egypt, recognized they would need water to exist, therefore they constructed their cities next to rivers. They made use of water for farming, cooking, drinking, and even sacred rituals.

As we move forward in time, scientists have discovered even more reasons why water is so crucial. Researchers have found that maintaining proper hydration can enhance focus, emotional stability, and even physical performance. We'll speak about the risks of dehydration next, which is another lesson from modern science.

However, we must not overlook the knowledge of our forefathers. They respected water because they understood that it held the key to life. Although we now have the means to clean and safe-for-drinking water, the essential need for water doesn't change.

1.3 Dehydration: The Covert Danger Inside

When your body doesn't have enough water to function correctly, it becomes dehydrated. It resembles when a plant begins to wilt from not receiving enough water. You may experience symptoms such as fatigue, headaches, dizziness, and thirst when you're dehydrated.

However, feeling thirsty isn't the only sign of dehydration. Because sometimes you're not aware of how much it's hurting you, it poses a silent threat. Water is essential for both your body and brain to function at their peak, and dehydration can make it difficult to focus and maintain energy. It's like attempting to run a race without any fuel.

Dehydration that is severe enough can be fatal. It may potentially be fatal and cause heat stroke and kidney issues. Water consumption is therefore crucial throughout the day, particularly in hot weather and during physical activity.

1.4 What Makes Water? Examining Its Special Qualities

When you think about it, water is actually rather fantastic. It is ideal for supporting life because of a few special qualities. These are a handful:

1. Solvent Power: Water is referred to be the "universal solvent" due to its exceptional ability to dissolve a wide range of compounds. This implies that it can transport chemicals, minerals, and nutrients to the areas of your body where they are required. It functions like a superhero, supplying every region of your body with necessities.

2.

3. Temperature Regulation: Adding water to your body can assist control its temperature. Your body sweats, largely consisting of water, when it gets hot. You

become cooler as the perspiration on your skin evaporates. It resembles the internal air cooling system of your body.

4.

5. Lubrication and Cushioning: Water serves as a lubricant and cushion in your eyes, joints, and spinal cord. This safeguards your important organs and keeps your movements fluid. Water acts as a cushion inside your body, providing the same kind of protection from shocks and bumps.

6.

7. Chemical processes: Watery environments are the site of several chemical processes that are necessary for your survival. Water aids in the digestion of food so that your body can use it as fuel. It functions similarly to the secret component in a recipe that brings everything together.

8.

9. Transportation: Blood circulation depends on water. Blood, which is primarily composed of water, carries nutrients and oxygen to cells while also eliminating waste. It functions as the delivery and garbage trucks of your body, ensuring that everything is delivered to

its proper location and remaining tidy.

Water is not merely significant—it is vital. It is the fundamental component of our body, has been prized since antiquity, and is supported by contemporary research. Although dehydration is a quiet danger, we can recognize its vital role in maintaining our health and well-being by comprehending the special qualities of water. So, to keep your body happy and hydrated, remember to drink lots of water every day!

CHAPTER 2

HYDRATION'S SYMPHONY: ADVANTAGES FOR ALL SYSTEMS

2.1 Brainpower Boost: How Hydration Enhances Cognitive Function

Consider the human brain to be a supercomputer. This supercomputer requires water as a unique fuel to function at its peak! Water consumption keeps your mind clear and attentive. Insufficient alcohol consumption might cause disorientation and make it difficult to concentrate in class.

Water facilitates improved communication between brain cells. Consider it analogous to the oil that maintains a machine's smooth operation. Your brain's cells can transmit and receive information more effectively if they are properly hydrated. This translates into increased mental speed, improved memory, and ease of problem-solving.

Water also contributes to a balanced mood. You may have irritability or fatigue if you're dehydrated. You can feel happier and more energized if you drink enough water. So, to help you get back on track when you're feeling a little off, try having a glass of water!

2.2 The Digestive Dance: The Function of Water in Healthy Living

Your digestive tract breaks down food into nutrients that provide you energy and maintain your health, much like a conveyor belt transports food through your body. A crucial component of this process is water.

Water aids in the breakdown of food in the stomach during eating. It would be difficult to try to wash muck off your hands without any water, don't you think? Water facilitates the conversion of food into a form that is easily absorbed and utilized by the body.

Water facilitates food passage through the intestines as well. The conveyor belt slows down and you may become constipated if you don't drink enough water, which makes it difficult to use the restroom. As oil keeps gears turning, drinking plenty of water keeps everything running smoothly.

2.3 Water and Skin Health: Radiant from the Inside Out

The largest organ in your body, your skin requires water to keep hydrated and radiant. Consider your skin to be a sponge. It is pliable and supple when properly hydrated. It can get flaky, tight, and dry if it doesn't get enough water.

Water consumption keeps your skin hydrated from the inside out. It clears the body of toxins, or bad material, which can accumulate and lead to skin issues like acne. Additionally, water helps your skin cells absorb nutrients, which strengthens and improves their health.

Your skin can appear more radiant and brighter when you consume enough water. It's similar to watering a plant; given enough water, it can develop into a robust, lovely plant. Thus, make sure you drink enough water each day to maintain the best-looking skin.

2.4 Maintaining the Engine: Water and Physical Capacity

Your body functions similarly to a high-performance machine, and like any machine, it requires the proper fuel to operate properly. That fuel contains a lot of water. Maintaining proper hydration is essential for your body to function at its peak, whether you're engaging in physical activity, playing sports, or just going about your everyday business.

Your body begins to sweat to relieve the heat produced by your working muscles. Since sweat is primarily made up of water, dehydration can occur if you don't replenish the water lost through perspiration. You may experience muscle cramps as well as fatigue and sluggishness as a result of this.

Water also improves the function of your muscles. You can move more quickly and powerfully when your muscles are well-hydrated because they can contract more readily. It's similar to having smoothly rotating, noise-free, well-oiled gears.

Water also aids in the prevention of injuries. Joints and muscles that are well-hydrated are more flexible and less likely to sprain or strain. If you drink enough water, your body will remain flexible and ready for action, much like a rubber band that is stretchable without breaking.

Water is necessary for all bodily systems. It boosts your brainpower, helps your digestive system run smoothly, keeps your skin healthy, and enhances your physical performance. Just like a symphony needs all its instruments to play in harmony, your body needs water to function at its best. So, remember to drink plenty of water every day to keep the symphony of hydration playing beautifully in your body!

CHAPTER 3

PAY ATTENTION TO YOUR BODY: IDENTIFYING DEHYDRATION SIGNS

3.1 The Thirst Trap: The Reasons Why You Don't Feel Wet All the Time

Consider the human body as a large, active factory. Similar to the oil that keeps all the machinery operating properly is water. However, the factory may not always indicate when extra oil is required. The "thirst trap" is that.

Your body uses thirst as a signal to tell you, "Hey, I need more water!" However, sometimes, particularly when you're engrossed in an enjoyable activity, you could miss the signs of thirst until you're starting to feel a little dehydrated. This implies that your body needs water even before you experience thirst.

Consider it akin to an automobile. You risk getting stranded on the side of the road if you wait to fill up the gas tank until it is empty. It is preferable to keep it filled. Similar to this, maintaining a regular water intake—even when you're not thirsty—helps your body function properly.

3.2 Beyond Thirst: Dehydration's Physical Symptoms

Being dehydrated is more than just being thirsty. Your body may give you a lot more indications that it needs extra water. Let's examine a few of these:

- Dry Mouth and Lips: You need to drink more water if your lips are chapped or your mouth feels dry.
- Dark Yellow Urine: Light yellow pee indicates dehydration. You should drink more water if it's amber or dark yellow.
- Fatigue: Excessive fatigue may indicate dehydration. There isn't enough water in your body to sustain your energy levels.
- Headaches: Your body may be dehydrated if you have headaches.
- Dizziness: Dehydration might cause you to feel lightheaded or dizzy. For your brain to work

correctly, it needs water.

- Dry Skin: You need additional water if your skin feels less elastic or dry.

It's critical to identify these symptoms and sip water before experiencing extreme thirst. Your body is similar to a plant in that it needs frequent irrigation to remain robust and healthy.

3.3 The Body-Mind Link: Hydration and Cognitive Impairment

Your brain functions as your body's command center. For optimal performance, it requires water. You cannot have proper brain function while you are dehydrated. This is referred to as cognitive decline, which is just a fancy term for when your brain isn't functioning as it should.

Concentration might be difficult when dehydrated. Your brain feels as though it is dehydrated when you attempt to complete your assignments while you are extremely exhausted. You may also experience difficulties with problem-solving or memory.

Your mood might also be impacted by dehydration. Not getting enough water could make you grumpy or more easily agitated. Rehydrating your brain facilitates pleasant, clear thinking.

3.4 The Ripple Effect of Dehydration: Its Effect on Other Health Conditions

One thing can lead to another like a domino effect when dehydrated. Insufficient water consumption can exacerbate other health issues. Let's examine a few instances:

- Kidney Stones: Waste products are removed from your blood by your kidneys. Kidney stones may result from dehydration because there is not enough water in the body to adequately break down waste. These hurt and may lead to major health problems.

- Digestive Issues: Your digestive system cannot function correctly if you don't drink enough water. Constipation from this may make it difficult to urinate.

- High Blood Pressure: When you're dehydrated, your

blood might thicken and become more difficult for your heart to pump. Your blood pressure may rise as a result, which is bad for your heart.

- Joint Pain: To keep your joints lubricated, water is necessary. If you don't drink enough water, you may become stiff or have joint pain.

Adequate hydration aids in averting these issues and maintains optimal bodily functions. Similar to routine auto maintenance, it keeps everything in working order and averts more serious problems later on.

Staying hydrated and paying attention to your body are essential for maintaining good health. Dehydration can be indicated by a variety of physical symptoms in addition to thirst. Dehydration has an impact on your body, mind, and emotions. It may also exacerbate pre-existing medical ailments, leading to a cascade of issues. Thus, to feel your best every day, don't forget to stay hydrated and drink enough water!

CHAPTER 4

SELECTING THE APPROPRIATE DRINKS TO QUENCH YOUR THIRST SENSATIONS

4.1 Plain Water: The Unchallenged Winner

Envision yourself engaging in an extended, enjoyable game. You need the best fuel to keep performing at your best, and plain water is that fuel for your body. Because it contains no additional substances that could cause you to slow down, water is like a superhero for your body. It is pure and just what your body requires to maintain proper hydration.

Your organs, muscles, and cells function best when you drink plain water. It is the healthiest option because it has no calories, sugar, or caffeine. You're providing the best possible nutrition for your body each time you take a sip. It's similar to selecting the highest caliber components for your beloved toy to ensure years of flawless operation.

Thus, it's always a good idea to go for a glass of water

when you're thirsty. It's what your body most desires since it's pure, uncomplicated, and simple!

4.2 Flavored Waters: Infusing Adventure and Taste

It's acceptable if plain water seems a touch monotonous at times. You can add natural tastes to make it more fascinating. This is known as infused water, and it tastes just like you're adding something delicious to your water without adding anything bad.

Slices of cucumber, oranges, lemons, strawberries, and even vegetables can be added. Herbs in season, such as basil or mint, can further enhance the flavor of your water. Imagine your water changing into a delightful, vibrant beverage that has all the advantages of regular water plus some exciting new flavors.

If you find ordinary water to be a little boring, infused waters are a terrific way to stay hydrated. It's also a great chance to try out several flavors and discover which ones you prefer. It's similar to creating a sundae with your preferred toppings out of an ordinary ice cream cone!

4.3 Interpreting Drinks: Knowing Sugar- and Caffeine-Induced Drinks

Not every beverage is made equally. Certain beverages, such as energy drinks and sodas, are high in caffeine and sugar. Although some beverages taste wonderful, your body may not react well to them.

- Sugary Drinks: Sugar content is high in soda, fruit punches, and sweetened teas. Even while they could provide you with a little energy boost, the effects are fleeting and can wear you out later. It's like a sugar rush. In addition, eating too much sugar can lead to weight gain and dental problems. Like eating too many candies at once, it may be enjoyable in the short term but is bad for you in the long run.

-

- Caffeinated Drinks: Caffeine is an ingredient in tea, coffee, and energy drinks. Although too much caffeine can cause jitters and anxiety, it is a stimulant that can help you feel more awake. Caffeine doesn't truly help youngsters focus or get a good night's sleep; in fact, it can make these things more difficult. It can cause the car to run too fast and crash, just like when you put too much gas in an automobile.

It's critical to read labels and be aware of the ingredients in your beverages. Drinking beverages low in sugar and caffeine is always a better method to stay hydrated and healthy.

4.4 Electrolytes Expounded: Their Significance

Perhaps you've heard about electrolytes in sports drinks and have been curious about their nature. Minerals called electrolytes, such as calcium, potassium, and sodium, aid in maintaining the proper balance of bodily fluids. They are essential for maintaining the health of your nerves and muscles.

Excessive exercise, particularly on warm days, causes you to perspire and lose electrolytes and water. That's when electrolyte-containing beverages, such as sports drinks, might assist in making up for what you've lost. But for regular activity, you can generally stay hydrated with just simple water.

Sports drinks are recommended for prolonged periods of intense exertion, such as a marathon or several hours of soccer play. However, keep in mind that a lot of sports drinks also contain additional sugars, making them a poor option for everyday hydration. Like specialized tools that are only needed for certain tasks, simple water works just fine most of the time.

Selecting the appropriate drinks is critical to maintaining good health and adequate hydration. The greatest option is plain water since it is pure and just what your body needs. Without adding any unhealthy additions, infused waters can offer a unique touch. Drinks high in sugar and caffeine should be used with caution as they may have negative effects on your health. Recall that while electrolytes are beneficial during vigorous exercise, they are not always required. Thus, use the greatest hydration options to maintain your body functioning properly and effectively quench your thirst!

CHAPTER 5

5.1 Customize Your Hydration: Determine Your Daily Requirements

Water is necessary for everyone, yet not everyone requires the same amount. Similar to how certain plants require more water than others. Determining your daily water requirements is crucial and is influenced by factors such as age, weight, level of activity, and even the climate.

Here's a quick method to estimate how much water you require: It's customary to have eight 8-ounce glasses of water every day. It's called the "8x8 rule." But depending on what you require, this can alter. For instance, you'll need more water if you're playing outside on a hot day because you'll be perspiring more.

To determine how much water you need, you can also use

your weight. Half your body weight in pounds should be consumed in ounces of water. Therefore, you should try to drink roughly 30 ounces of water a day if you weigh 60 pounds. That is equivalent to consuming roughly four normal water bottles.

5.2 Establish a Habit: Easy Ways to Remain Hydrated During the Day

If you incorporate staying hydrated into your everyday routine, it can be simple to maintain. The following straightforward methods will assist you in remembering to drink water:

- Start Your Day with Water: As soon as you wake up, have a glass of water to start your day. It helps you wake up and feels like a fresh start for your body.
- Have a Water Bottle: Whether you're at home relaxing or participating in sports, make sure you always have a water bottle with you. In this manner, water will always be close at hand for when you get thirsty.
- Set Reminders: Make a note to yourself or on your

phone or watch to remember to drink water on a regular basis. You're merely reminding yourself to take care of your body, just like when you set an alarm to remind you to feed your pet.

- Drink Water with Meals: Develop the practice of sipping a glass of water before, during, and after every meal. It keeps you hydrated and aids in improved food digestion.

- Taste Your Water: If you think plain water is boring, liven it up with some fruit slices or a squeeze of juice. This can add flavor and pleasure to drinking water.

5.3 Technology to the Rescue: Apps and Notifications to Help You Stay Hydrated

Our world is filled with amazing technological advancements that can assist us with nearly anything, including drinking water! Numerous devices and apps are available that are intended to keep you hydrated. Here are some suggestions:

- Hydration Apps: You can keep track of how much

water you drink with the help of apps like "Plant Nanny" or "Hydro Coach." Not only can these applications remind you to stay hydrated, but they can also make it an enjoyable game where you have to water a virtual plant in order to keep it alive.

- Smart Water Bottles: Certain water bottles have integrated notifications or lights that indicate when it's time to drink. They are even able to monitor your daily water intake.

- Alarm Clocks and Timers: Use your phone or watch's alarm or timer feature to remind you to sip water once an hour. It's an easy method to make sure you're continuing on your current course.

Staying hydrated can be more enjoyable and easy when you use technology. It serves as a reminder to look after oneself, much like having a personal coach.

5.4 Have Fun and Taste: Concoctions for Delectably Refreshing Drinks

It's acceptable for plain water to occasionally become monotonous! You may stay hydrated and content by making delectable and healthful drinks at home. Here are a few simple recipes to try:

- Citrus Splash: In a pitcher of water, add slices of orange, lime, and lemon. Give it some time to settle so the flavors can meld. It tastes just like delicious lemonade without all the added sugar!

- Berry Blast: Incorporate frozen or fresh berries into your water, such as raspberries, blueberries, and strawberries. The berries will provide a delightfully tart and sweet flavor.

- Cucumber Mint Cooler: Incorporate some fresh mint leaves and cucumber slices into your water. This beverage is very cooling, particularly in the summer.

- Watermelon Water: Process watermelon chunks with a squeeze of lime juice and a little water. This produces a naturally sweet, refreshing beverage that is ideal for summer.

- Herbal Iced Tea: Pour your preferred herbal tea into a mug and let it cool. For a caffeine-free beverage that is both refreshing and hydrating, add ice and a slice of lemon.

These recipes add flavor and excitement to plain water. Try experimenting with various fruits and herbs to discover your best pairings.

It's critical for your health to be hydrated, and there are lots of enjoyable and simple ways to make sure you drink enough water. Determine how much water you need on a personal basis, utilize technology to help you remember, develop a habit of drinking it, and experiment with tasty recipes to keep things fresh. These hydration tips can help you stay energized and prepared for all of your travels!

CHAPTER 6

EXERCISE-RELATED HYDRATION: FUELING YOUR FITNESS

6.1 Hydration is Key to Optimal Performance Before Exercise

It's similar to preparing your body for a major journey before you begin any exercise or participate in sports. Making sure you're hydrated is among the most crucial things you can do. Water consumption prior to exercise maintains your energy levels and improves the function of your muscles.

Here's a basic guideline: Aim for roughly 16 ounces (2 cups) of water two hours before beginning an exercise regimen. This allows your body adequate time to prepare for action by absorbing the water. Similar to refueling your car before a lengthy road trip, you want to get off to a full tank!

It's acceptable if you work out first thing in the morning or if you neglect to hydrate beforehand! To ensure that you are not dehydrated before your workout, simply take tiny sips of water beforehand.

6.2 Rehydrating While Exercising: Techniques to Prevent Dehydration

You perspire to keep cool while you run about or perform sports. You risk becoming dehydrated if you don't replenish the water lost via sweat. Here's how to drink enough water when working out:

1. Drink Before You're Thirsty: You're already beginning to become dehydrated by the time you experience thirst. For this reason, even if you don't feel thirsty yet, consistently drink tiny sips of water.
2.
3. Sports Drinks: Sports drinks with electrolytes can help replenish what you lose via sweat if you're engaging in vigorous exercise for longer than an hour, such as playing soccer or running a race.
4. These beverages improve muscle function and provide you with energy.

5.

6. Water Breaks: Throughout your exercise, take brief breaks to sip water or a sports drink. Similar to taking a breather, you're providing your body with the nourishment it needs to continue operating at full capacity.

7.

8. Pay Attention to Your Body: You may need to drink additional water if you begin to feel lightheaded, exhausted, or have a dry mouth. Your body is communicating with you like a perceptive buddy; learn to read its signals!

6.3 Rehydration Is Crucial for Post-Workout Recovery

Following physical activity, your body requires rest and replenishment. Drinking water to replenish what you lost via perspiration is part of this. This is the reason it matters:

- Muscle Recovery: Water consumption speeds up the body's natural healing process after exercise. It's similar to offering them a cool beverage to aid with relaxation and strength-building.

- Cool Down: Your body retains heat after physical activity. Similar to sipping a cold beverage on a hot day, drinking water makes you feel cooler from the inside out.

- Replace Electrolytes: You may have lost electrolytes such as potassium and sodium if you have been perspiring a lot. You can replenish them by eating an electrolyte-containing snack or drinking a sports drink.

Are you thirsty? Cheers!: Water consumption is vital after exercise, even if you don't feel very thirsty. In order to keep you feeling well and prepared for your next excursion, your body needs to replenish the fluids that it lost.

6.4 Hydration Needs-Based on Exercise Type: Particular Requirements for Various Workouts

The requirements for hydration vary depending on the kind of exercise. Here's how to customize your water intake:

- Endurance Sports (like Cycling or Running): You'll need to hydrate with water or a sports drink throughout these activities because they involve a lot of sweating.

- Strength Training (like Weightlifting): Drink plenty of water to keep your muscles functioning properly and avoid cramping, even though you may not be perspiring as much.

- Team sports (such as basketball or soccer): These contests require a lot of sprinting and quick reflexes. In order to stay hydrated and maintain a high level of energy, drink water or sports drinks.

- Yoga or Stretching: Your body still needs water to stay flexible and maintain the health of your joints, even if you're not sprinting around. Drink water both before and after your workout.

Recall that each kind of exercise is like a unique game with its own set of rules. You may keep hydrated and perform at your best by sipping water or sports drinks appropriate for the kind of exercise you're performing.

Maintaining proper hydration when exercising is crucial to maintaining the strength and health of your body. To assist your muscles recover from exercise, consume water before you begin, during your workout, and afterward. Make sure to select the appropriate drinks for your training regimen as different forms of activity have varied hydration requirements. You'll be prepared to take on any challenge and remain at the top of your game with these pointers!

CHAPTER 7

7.1 Establishing Healthful Routines: Adequate Hydration for Kids and Teens

Hi there! For kids and teens like you, staying hydrated is crucial whether you're playing games, studying hard, or just having fun. This is the reason why:

- Expanding Bodies: Water promotes the healthy and robust growth of all the parts of your body that are always changing and expanding. Giving your body the nutrition it needs to keep developing like a superhero is what it feels like!

- Energy Boost: Whether you're concentrating in class or rushing around at recess, drinking water keeps you energized throughout the day.

- Learning and Concentration: Drinking water improves brain function, which enables you to

34

absorb and retain new information. It's similar to having a smart juice that makes everything you do better.

Try to consume water throughout the day to stay hydrated. When playing outside, carry a water bottle with you or keep one on hand. Keep in mind that your body still requires water to function properly even if you don't feel thirsty.

7.2 Retaining Vitality: Adult Requirements for Hydration

Even as you become older, your body still requires a lot of water to be strong and healthy. Adults should stay hydrated for the following reasons:

- Daily Functioning: Water supports healthy muscle and organ function, enabling you to engage in all of your favorite activities, including working out, going to work, and socializing with loved ones.
- Healthy Skin: Maintaining enough hydration levels maintains your skin smooth and radiant. It is like

providing your skin with a cooling beverage from the inside out.

- Digestive Health: Drinking water facilitates a healthy digestive tract that allows you to absorb all the nutrients from food and digest it.

Strive to consume eight glasses of water or more each day to stay hydrated. If you're exercising frequently or it's extremely hot outside, you might need extra. To remind yourself to drink frequently, carry a water bottle with you to work or on errands.

7.3 Aging Gracefully: Seniors' Need for Hydration

Our bodies alter as we age, but maintaining enough hydration is still crucial. This is why elders need to stay hydrated:

- Joint Health: Water helps lubricate your joints, allowing for easier and more comfortable movement.
- Cognitive Function: Hydration aids in memory and focus by supporting brain function. It's similar to giving your mind the replenishment it requires to

remain sharp.

- Heart and Kidney Health: Drinking water supports healthy blood circulation and waste removal in the kidneys. It's similar to providing these vital organs with support to maintain their health.

Drink water all throughout the day to stay hydrated. Even though we may not feel as thirsty as we once did as we age, our bodies still require water. To remind yourself to stay hydrated, always have a bottle or glass of water handy, especially if you take any medications that may cause dehydration.

7.4 Extra Care: Staying Hydrated Throughout Pregnancy and Breastfeeding

It's important for new and expectant mothers to stay hydrated for the sake of both you and your child. The following explains why it's crucial to stay hydrated whether pregnant or nursing:

- Development of the Baby: Water aids in the formation of the placenta and amniotic fluid throughout pregnancy, giving your unborn child a healthy environment in which to thrive.

- Milk Production: Getting adequate water helps nursing mothers produce enough milk to give their babies the nutrition they require.
- Health of Moms: Drinking enough water helps avoid constipation, exhaustion, and other typical pregnancy and lactation discomforts.

Drink a lot of water throughout the day to stay hydrated. When you're pregnant or nursing, try to drink at least 10 glasses of water per day. Carry a water bottle with you at all times, and sip from it when you're feeling peckish or after nursing your child.

Feeling your best is mostly dependent on being hydrated, regardless of your stage of life. Water is essential for growth and learning in children and teenagers, daily living and healthy skin in adults, joint and brain health in elderly, and pregnancy and lactation in mothers, who require extra hydration. Thus, enjoy your drink and maintain a happy, healthy body at any age!

CHAPTER 8

DISPELLING MYTHS ABOUT HYDRATION AND DIFFERENTIATING REAL FROM FICTION

8.1 The Magic Number in the 8-Glass Rule: Is It There?

You may have heard that in order to maintain good health, you should consume precisely eight glasses of water each day. But hey, what do you know? No single magic number works for everyone! Your age, weight, and level of activity will all affect how much water you require.

1. Listen to Your Body: Focus on your body rather than counting glasses. As soon as you feel thirsty, sip water. Your body can warn you when it needs water, much like an intelligent alarm clock.

2. Variety Matters: Consuming produce also replenishes your water intake. Therefore, you may not require as much plain water if you consume a lot of juicy fruits like oranges or watermelon.

3. Remain in Balance: Sip water all day long. You'll need extra if you're physically active or it's hot outside. It's similar to filling up your gas tank in that you require more gasoline (water) the more you drive or play.

8.2 Is It Possible to Over Hydrate? Recognizing Acid-Base Imbalance

Although you may believe that consuming a lot of water is always beneficial, is there ever too much? You certainly can! Your body's equilibrium may be thrown off if you drink too much water without also consuming enough food or replenishing electrolytes (such potassium and sodium).

1. Electrolytes Are Important: These minerals support the proper function of your muscles, nerves, and other bodily parts. They can become diluted by excessive water consumption, which can lead to issues like headaches, nausea, and in severe situations, seizures.

2. Staying in Balance: Pay attention to your body. You might not immediately require more water if you're not thirsty. It's similar to eating; you want the perfect quantity, neither too much nor too little.

3. Moderation Is Best: You may maintain your body's equilibrium by eating a balanced diet that includes fruits, vegetables, and some salty snacks (such pretzels or almonds) as well as drinking water when you're thirsty.

8.3 Water-Based Detoxification: Real or Illusion?

It's possible that you've heard that drinking a lot of water aids in the body's detoxification process. The good news is that your body already has an excellent detoxification system! Your kidneys and liver put forth a lot of effort to remove waste and maintain your health.

1. Water Helps Your Organs: By supporting your liver and kidneys, drinking water can help them function more effectively. It's akin to giving them a high five for continuing to perform well.

2. No Quick Fixes: Your body won't magically get cleansed by drinking water on its own. The greatest methods to assist your body's natural detoxification process are to maintain an active lifestyle and eat a balanced diet rich in fruits and vegetables.

3. Healthy Habits: Make drinking water a regular part of your day rather than concentrating on "detox" diets or beverages. Your body is capable of healing itself!

8.4 Dispelling Frequently Held Myths About Water vs. Other Drinks

While water is wonderful, what about other beverages? Let's dispel a few myths:

- Sugary Drinks: Sugar-filled beverages, such as soda and juices with added sweeteners, can cause tooth decay and weight gain. It's similar to overindulging in candy—fun at first, but ultimately unhealthy.

- Caffeinated Drinks: Caffeine, which is present in tea and coffee, can help you feel awake but, if consumed in excess, can cause jitters and difficulty falling asleep. Children often don't require caffeine.

- Healthy Choices: Since water is healthy for your body and has no calories or sugar, it's the best option for staying hydrated. A delicious spin on water can be achieved by adding fruits or herbs if you're looking for something flavorful.

Though you should occasionally enjoy other beverages, water is the most beneficial beverage for your body's overall wellbeing. So go ahead and remain hydrated by sticking to the simple, revitalizing option of water!

Being aware of hydration myths enables you to choose your beverages wisely. There is no magic amount of water that you should consume; instead, pay attention to your body. Moderation is crucial since drinking too much water without eating enough might throw off your body's equilibrium. Water helps your body's natural detoxification process, but there are no shortcuts. Water is the best option, but other liquids are OK in moderation. Maintain proper hydration to keep your body in peak condition!

CHAPTER 9

ECO-CONSCIOUS HYDRATION FOR A SUSTAINABLE FUTURE

9.1 Bottled water's Effect on the Environment: A Change Request

Hi there! Unbeknownst to you, bottled water might have a significant negative environmental impact. This is the reason why:

1. Plastic Problem: Plastic bottles are used to package most bottled water. The production of these bottles consumes a lot of energy and oil. It can take hundreds of years for them to decompose after being thrown away, and some wind up in the ocean and harm marine life.

2. Transportation Costs: Trucks that produce pollution and exacerbate climate change are frequently used to transport bottled water across great distances to retail locations.

3. Waste Issues: Although plastic bottles are recyclable, a large number of them wind up in landfills. It's the equivalent of discarding something that might still be helpful!

9.2 Reusable Bottles: Choosing Eco-Friendly

Try using a reusable container that you can fill with water from your house or a water fountain in place of single-use plastic bottles. This is why it's a really good idea:

Environmentally Friendly: Since reusable bottles may be filled and reused repeatedly, less new plastic bottles are needed. It's similar like being able to play with your favorite toy every day!

Saves Money: Over time, purchasing bottled water can add up. Reusable bottles assist your family's finances by saving money.

Personalized Style: You can pick a bottle that embodies your own style, such as one colored in your favorite hue or adorned with amusing stickers!

9.3 Filtering at Home: An Affordable and Sustainable Choice

Try using a water filter if you want pure, delicious water at home without having to purchase bottled water. This is why it's fantastic:

1. Clean Water: Tap water is made to taste great and fresh by filtering out contaminants and undesirable tastes. It's similar to turning regular water into something exceptional!

2. Less Waste: Rather than purchasing bottled water, you can use a filter to fill your reusable bottle with tap water. This benefits the environment and cuts down on plastic trash.

3. Cost Savings: Over time, filters are less expensive than purchasing a large quantity of bottled water. It's similar to putting money aside for a fun project rather of splurging on a one-time purchase.

9.4 Water Conservation: Minor Actions, Major Effects

Conserving water is good for the environment as well. Here's how you can contribute:

Turn Off Taps: Shut off the faucet when not in use, such as when you brush your teeth or wash your hands. A lot of water is saved!

- Shorter Showers: Less water is used when taking shorter showers. Try setting a time limit for yourself to see how fast you can clean up!

- Fix Leaks: Report to an adult so they can fix any leaks you find in the toilet or tap. Every drop matters!

- Outdoor Watering: Water plants with a watering bucket rather than a hose. It conserves water and is more accurate.

You may contribute to the preservation of our planet by

using water wisely at home and using environmentally friendly products like water filters and reusable bottles. A small action taken over time can have a significant impact!

Being environmentally responsible when it comes to hydration entails making wise decisions that benefit the ecosystem. Reusable bottles are preferable to single-use ones when it comes to transportation. For a waste-free, fresh flavor, consider filtering your own water at home. And never forget that conserving water is simple and crucial—every drop matters! By working together, we can build a sustainable future where a healthy world and pure water coexist.

10.1 Make an Investment in Your Health: Hydration Is Essential for Long-Term Health

Hi there! Taking care of your body is similar to caring for a unique plant since both require water to flourish and remain healthy. This is why maintaining proper hydration is crucial for your long-term health:

1. Body Balance: Getting adequate water into your body makes it function as one cohesive unit, much like a well-oiled machine. It maintains your brain, muscles, and organs in peak condition.

2. Avoiding Issues: Drinking enough water helps avoid headaches, fatigue, and even more serious conditions like renal difficulties. It is comparable to applying sunscreen to prevent skin burns.

3. Healthy Habits: You're putting yourself on the path to a lifetime of good health by forming the habit of drinking water now. It is comparable to constructing a solid foundation for a sturdy home!

10.2 The Hydration Ripple Effect: Motivating Others to Drink Water

By taking care of yourself and drinking water, you encourage others to follow suit. Your actions can have the following cascading effects:

- Set an Example: Your loved ones may wish to follow suit if they observe you sipping water and seeming content. It's similar like igniting a wave of wholesome routines!

- Sharing is Caring: You can motivate people to drink water by explaining the value of being hydrated. Perhaps you'll get a thank-you for making them feel better!

- Healthy Community: Our entire community is happier and healthier when everyone drinks water and stays hydrated. It's similar to sports teamwork in that everyone participates!

10.3 Honor Your Achievements: Acknowledging Advancements on Your Hydration Path

It's crucial to recognize and honor the healthy habits you have, such as consistently consuming adequate water. Here's how to acknowledge your accomplishments:

- Set Goals: Choose a daily water intake target and monitor your progress. Celebrate when you reach your objective! It's similar to winning a race: you succeeded!

- Reward Yourself: Give yourself a treat when you accomplish goals, such as a week of consistent water consumption. It is comparable to receiving a gold star for your efforts.

- Remain Upbeat: Don't worry if you forget to drink

water one day. There's a fresh opportunity to attempt every day. Similar to training for a sport, practice makes perfect!

10.4 Live a Hydrated and Healthful Life by Embracing the Power of Water

Water has so many health benefits for your body, it's incredible! Here's how to use water's power in your daily life:

- Remain Energized: Water helps you stay energized so you can play, learn, and enjoy yourself all day long. It's akin to possessing an endless supply of strength!

- Healthy Skin: Drinking water keeps your skin radiant and clear. It's like applying a cool mist to your face to feel and look your best.

- Be Your Best: Hydration improves your ability to move, think, and feel in general. It helps you overcome any obstacle like a secret weapon.

Recall that drinking water is a lifelong habit rather than something you do sometimes. You're putting yourself in a position to have a healthy and happy future by prioritizing your hydration, encouraging others, acknowledging your accomplishments, and harnessing the power of water. Be sure to stay hydrated and keep up the good work!

ABOUT THE AUTHOR

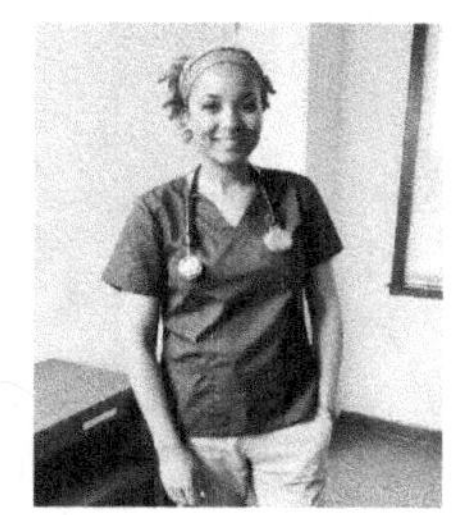 Harmony Royce is a dedicated healthcare worker who has a strong interest in holistic wellness. Harmony's extensive history in various aspects of health and wellness provides her with a wealth of knowledge and expertise that she can utilize in her writing and professional endeavors.

Harmony is a talented author who crafts thought-provoking books that inspire readers to have well-rounded, balanced lives. She writes about a variety of health-related topics, such as diet, exercise, mental health, and mindfulness. Her approachable writing style combines practical guidance with evidence-based research to make complex health concepts approachable and engaging for readers of all ages.

Harmony actively promotes the benefits of holistic health through writing, community workshops, and internet forums. Her mission is to educate and inspire people about the transformative power of self-care and healthy lifestyle choices.

www.ingramcontent.com/pod-product-compliance
Lightning Source LLC
Chambersburg PA
CBHW051659250726
48653CB00007B/2754